HOW TO OVERCOME HEART DISEASE

Published by SAGAX Publishing
www.keithfoster.co.uk

Copyright © Keith Foster – July 2016

ISBN 978-0-9956128-0-8

A catalogue record for this book is available from the British Library

Keith Foster's right to be identified as the author of this work has been asserted by him in accordance with the Copyright, Designs and Patents Act of 1988.

Manufacture / Printing coordinated in the UK by
LightningSource.com

All rights reserved. No part of this book may be reproduced or transmitted in any form, electronic or mechanical, including photocopy or any information storage and retrieval system, without permission in writing from the publisher.

Disclaimer

This publication is for information only and should not be used for the diagnosis or treatment of health conditions. If you are ill or have a medical condition first consult a qualified doctor or specialist.

Dedication

To my father
Donald Edward Foster (1912 – 1949)
who died of heart disease and
who I've missed these last 66 years.

Other titles by Keith Foster

The Answer to Cancer. ISBN 978-0-9532407-5-3 (2016)

SUPER SLIM. ISBN 978-0-9532407-6-0

Harmonic Power Parts II – VI; ISBN 978-0-9532407-7-7

The Wisdom Way. ISBN 978-0-9532407-9-1

The Backball Method – *A Comprehensive Self-Help Guide to Back Pain Relief*. ISBN 978-0-9532407-2-2

Catastrophe – *A New Theory as to the Cause of Global Warming.* ISBN 978-0-9532407-3-9

Lifelight – *(How to protect yourself from cancer or help yourself if you get ill).* ISBN 978-0-9532407-1-5

Perfume, Astrology and You. ISBN 978-0-9532407-0-8

PREFACE

The purpose of this book is to provide you with information which will enable you to prevent heart disease or, if necessary, overcome it.

It contains new information which is derived from years of careful scientific research much of which was performed by intellectual giants such as Linus Pauling, the twice Nobel Laureate.

This is finally "capped off" by my own research into the electronic nature of life which was initiated both by personal tragedy, as I explained in the first two chapters, and by a need to arrive at an explanation for phenomena which could not otherwise be conceptualised.

In this book I talk a lot about Vitamin C and the reason for this is that some years ago I discovered that it has very special qualities which set it apart from other vitamins. Simply put, it is one of the building blocks of life which enabled energy transmission which enabled cells to transform into vigorous living structures and begin the long haul of evolution up to the present day.

In this book I describe the mechanism by which life uses Vitamin C and go on to illustrate this by demonstrating that our bodies simply begin to fall apart if we don't get enough of this marvellous substance.

I hope this helps you to "work up" your own self-treatment regime and in support of this I describe my daily dosages which, at age 75, have kept me healthy and illness free for the last 40 years.

I wish you good health.

Contents

Page Nos.

8. Chapter 1 - A Family Tragedy

15. Chapter 2 - Lean Times and Limeys
    Natural diet;

24. Chapter 3 - Scurvy
    The Linus Pauling video; Débâcle over cholesterol-lowering statin drugs; Transient global amnesia;

29. Chapter 4 - Further Proof
    Chronic scurvy verified by cardioretinometry and reversed with Vitamin C; Reversing coronary heart disease; Heal Yourself; Congenital heart defects and heart damage; Heart failure; High blood pressure/hypertension; Calcified arteries and osteoporosis; Heart attack;

35. Chapter 5 - The Beginning of Life on Earth
    Salts; Blood;

40. Chapter 6 - Vitamin C
    The Energy Bridge; Electron Transport; Essential Fuel for your immune system; About Vitamin C intake; The animal kingdom; How did this happen?; Vitamin C – an essential food; Hypoascorbemia; Self and not self;

51. Chapter 7 - Iodine
Fibrocystic Breast Disease; Seaweed; A Crucial Nutrient; Radiation Poisoning; Cheap & Nasty; Morbid Obesity;

57. Chapter 8 – Water
The Cholesterol Myth;

60. Chapter 9 – Obesity
Charcoal; C_{60} adds energy;

63. Chapter 10 - Charcoal
Adsorption; Rogue Oxygen Species; Rheology = Functional Shape;

67. Chapter 11 - How to Slow the Ageing Process
Magnetism & Earthing; Magnetic fields on health; The decline of the field; Diurnal Flow; Our new electronic environment; Boyers Binding Mechanism; How to Protect Yourself; The 'umbrella' effect; Earthing is dose related;

77. Chapter 12 - Moccasins and Magnets
Disconnecting; Natural Gait; Moccasins; Blood thinning; Inflammation & Ageing; Pain; Jet lag; Earthing;

85. My Daily Dosages.

88. Conclusion.

90. References.

Chapter 1

A Family Tragedy

When I was eight years old tragedy struck my family. My father died of a heart attack whilst at work.

It happened like this. There was an office party going on and it was Christmas Eve. He came out of his office into the general office where people were batting balloons around having drinks and generally enjoying themselves. Somebody batted a balloon toward him, he hit it with his right hand and collapsed dead on the floor. We were told that the large artery leading into his heart had furred up and that had stopped his heart beating.

The news arrived first over the telephone and then in person when one of his colleagues came to break it to my mother. She collapsed and then went the appalling ordeal of having to tell my brother and I and then having to organise a funeral of the man she idolised.

These events changed her personality when she became quite demented with grief and she was never the same again.

Meantime my brother and I were shut away in the sitting-room whilst all the neighbours and friends came in to commiserate with my mother.

My brother and I hadn't a clue what was going on and didn't in fact learn the truth until well into Christmas day, when we became confused and traumatised.

We didn't know our father well because I was born during the war and my father was away fighting. My brother was born just after the war and was four years younger than me, so knew father even less well.

As you can imagine this tragedy had very far reaching effects on what, up until that point, had been an ordinary middle-class family bringing up children and with great plans for their future.

My father had been a high achiever, having studied French at the Sorbonne in Paris before the war and had at the time of his death been a quite highly placed manager in a very-well run Quaker company in the north-east of England.

All this may seem very mundane to the reader, however, this is where the story really begins.

My father had been a weak child, one of three born to my grandpa and grandma who were an "old school" Victorian couple with a very strict set of values. My father had grown up learning the violin from grandpa and had achieved such skill with this instrument that he won prizes all over the county and ultimately played briefly with the Hallé Orchestra.

All this would lead anybody to believe that he was a very academic sort of person. However, this couldn't be further from the truth. Quite early in life he toughened up by playing tennis, squash, cricket and all the other games associated with his background and upbringing. Apparently, he was a demon squash player with very quick reflexes (which I later inherited) and became a champion in Yorkshire before the war.

Like so many of his generation, when war was declared he joined up as a volunteer and was posted to a night fighter squadron flying beaufighters where he did advanced training as a pilot. Unfortunately, he was colour blind and therefore couldn't qualify as a pilot being relegated to a staff job. This didn't suit him at all and as the war rolled on he applied for and joined a specialist unit being trained as commandos in Scotland.

From here on in the story gets a bit hazy, but we know that because of his French education (he was virtually bi-lingual, courtesy of a very pretty French lady I met years later). He was dropped into occupied France where he worked with the underground (the Maquis) in several different areas.

My father was dark-haired and lean and could have passed for a Frenchman anywhere.

It's not widely known, but prior to the Normandy landings, several intrepid "pathfinder" units were landed at nights on the Normandy coast and my father was amongst these, his role being to act as liaison between the Canadian divisions and the British Army on Sword Beach. Out of the 20 men in his unit who were landed he was the only survivor, although it was a close run thing and coincidence entered life here when under machine-gun fire he dived into a ditch which was already occupied by a wounded Canadian solider who had the same name as my father, Donald Foster. The poor Canadian chap who'd been machine gunned in the stomach died shortly after and my father made it back behind the lines.

He was then withdrawn to the UK when I was told he rather expected to be promoted and instead found himself being "volunteered" to be dropped into Denmark.

Why Denmark? Well, I should explain, that one branch of our family originated in Heligoland, an island in the German Bight, where Danish and German were spoken side by side until the late 20th century. Our Danish connections weren't strong, but father had distant relatives there whom he could contact and stay with monitoring the German withdrawal. As the Wehrmacht pulled back, under pressure from the Russian Army, they abandoned a great deal of kit and there's a photograph of my father sitting in the cockpit of an abandoned Heinkel on an airfield littered with perfectly serviceable planes that had had to be left behind.

I have no idea what service my father performed for our government or the Danish government, but he was later decorated by the Danes and given a silver signet ring which was apparently of some significance to the people in this area at this time. It's now proudly worn by my oldest son who is the very spitting image of my father, being dark and good looking.

As the war drew to a close, my father was repatriated to the UK bringing with him a rather handsome radiogram and several bottles of 'Cherry Heering' which were stamped for the use of the Luftwaffe only! Clearly these had been "liberated" from the defeated enemy, who, by that time, had withdrawn to Schleswig-Holstein and surrendered.

All of the foregoing begs the question, how is it that an extremely healthy, tough, athletic, highly motivated, vigorous man could possibly die of heart failure at an office party three years later. He didn't drink much, he smoked (but then everybody did during the war), he still played squash and tennis and was lean and fit. How is it then that he died of heart failure? This question has haunted me for 75 years and, because I believe I've found the answer, I've been boring you with all this family history as a run up to the revelation I intend to make to you. I sincerely hope it helps you as it has certainly helped me, so please read on.

CHAPTER 2

Lean times and Limeys

When I was a child and the war was raging on, there was universal food rationing in Britain and we were very nearly starving. Living close to the country and with relatives who had farms, we usually had enough to eat but it was often fairly poor stuff without much in the way of nutrition. The bread was grey and made up of all manner of different grains. Porridge was a staple and the meat ration of 8p, of 8 pennyworth a week was derisory. Pig clubs started up all over the land, rabbits were at a premium and pigeon and game birds were almost hunted out. As children, we fished the lakes and streams round about, went "chudding" which means raiding other people's orchards, set snares, grew everything we could in the garden and kept chickens.

I still remember the thrill of mushrooming in the ten acre field behind our house on a cold, damp September morning when the mist still clung to the earth. Wandering round in circles following the fairy rings, it was often quite funny to see the mist lift with the morning sun and find that you and 20 other neighbours were spread out across the field doing precisely the same thing. Little boys, old men and women out mushrooming (the men were all away at war). Hard times but with a great spirit of community.

During this time my father had it far worse, living on corned beef and whatever the Army and Airforce could scrape together to feed the men, a diet I might add which was almost totally devoid of any live food or any food containing much in the way of enzymes. And this is where the story begins because there's one vitamin missing from his diet and that lack has been responsible for more early deaths of heart disease than any war. What I'm talking about here is the relationship between Vitamin C deficiency and heart disease.

Pioneering research began in the late 1940s long after the structure of Vitamin C was determined when Canadian doctors proved that a Vitamin C deficiency causes the condition commonly called atherosclerosis. These researchers found that the condition will arise in 100% of

Vitamin C deprived animal test subjects that don't make their own Vitamin C.

Furthermore, these Canadian pioneers demonstrated that Vitamin C alone reverses atherosclerosis in laboratory animals. (G.C.Willis, "the reversibility of atherosclerosis" Canadian Medical Association Journal Volume 77 July 15th 1957, pages 106 to 109).

However, before getting into details of the modern cover up that's taken place, let's first look back at the origins of our knowledge in this field.

As naval technology advanced and shipwrights were able to build yet more efficient sailing ships, our ancestors took ever longer voyages of discovery.

Because half the time they didn't know where they were going, they often got lost or wandered off course or took prodigiously long times to progress to their various destinations. Because in those days food technology was very simple, i.e. food could be pickled, dried, salted or smoked. The ocean going diet was a very poor one. Ships loaded up with apples, livestock and vegetables but after they ran out, the diet became quite unpleasant with hardtack biscuits and salt fish or salt beef making up the most basic food regime.

Well into the second or third month of a long voyage, the crew started to become ill. This illness manifested itself in old wounds opening, appalling skin conditions, teeth falling out, eyesight failing and a whole range of ailments which are attendant on a poor diet.

Often these half crippled mariners would limp into port with well over half of their complement bedridden or dying and this, coupled with a lack of fresh water, was the scourge of all seafarers.

This general illness was called scurvy simply because skin flaked off people and their condition became what is now called scorbutic. However, a great change came about when in 1747 the naval physician, Dr. James Lind, first proposed that scurvy could be cured with oranges, limes and green vegetables. Like all pioneering medics he was ostracized by his colleagues for tainting the noble profession of medicine with worthless folklore.

It took another 48 years of evidence before the Royal Navy made limes a daily ration for British sailors and this is why we were called limeys by the Yanks who didn't share the same long distance voyages and therefore didn't suffer from scurvy half as badly as the British sailors.

The essential ingredient in limes, Vitamin C, was not isolated for another 133 years, in 1928, by the Nobel Prize winner, Albert Szent-Györgyi. Meantime, the use of citrus fruit slowly made its way through into the medical profession when it became firmly established as a treatment for scurvy.

The history of this kind of thing goes on endlessly in the medical profession. For example, at one time beriberi was also thought to be an infectious disease. When the Japanese researcher Kanehiro Takaki published evidence in the British Medical Journal Lancet in 1877 that diet could prevent beriberi he was ridiculed.

35 years later a biochemist, Casimir Funk, isolated the substance in rice husk that stops beriberi and this is the vitamin we now call thiamine.

It's the same old story, medical advances are made and poo-pooed by the establishment of the time. Then, the more sensible elements of this benighted profession begin to take on these ideas and within a time of around 50 years they are then incorporated into mainstream medicine. Curiously enough, around 50 years seems to be the time it takes for an idea to establish itself in a profession which prides itself on being founded on research and development and results!

This sad history continues today with pompous ridicule and an enormous lack of understanding before the acceptance of nutritional discoveries comes about. It's worth the mention in this context that, as of today, July 2016, the British Medical Association have just come round to the point of view that Vitamin D taken regularly in the winter can help people not only avoid rickets but also reduce a schedule of illnesses which heretofore had been treated with pharmaceutical drugs!

Natural diet

Until 10,000 years ago we were hunter gatherers foraging for our food which came from a wide range of sources. 83% of this was "green stuff", very rich in vitamins, particularly Vitamin C. The balance was protein which came from wild animals. Both the forage for the wild animals and the forage collected by our ancestors came from clean, nutrient-rich soil possessed of the 85 minerals required for optimum human health with no artificial additives, preservatives, dyes, emulsifiers and so forth. During this period human beings were the most healthy they've ever been as skeletal records show and this was the case until about 10,000 years ago when we started cultivating crops. The shift from a wide ranging diet over to monoculture of grains and the like had a profound effect on our species and new diseases began to emerge which were, to a certain extent, diet dependent.

However, the food was still grown on clean soil and because of the methods of crop rotation and returning manure to the land, fertility was kept high and our diets still contained the bulk of the vitamins and minerals that we need for optimum health.

Basically, this system of agriculture held sway until the late 18th century when the early development of nitrogenous fertilisers came into play.

So that the period during which long sea voyagers revealed the need for Vitamin C, runs alongside the fact that the bulk of the population were still getting plenty of minerals and vitamins from a diet grown on clean, healthy soils.

The change which has brought about the modern epidemic of scurvy has only come about in the last 100 years or so, so in a way the sailors who suffered appalling conditions of scurvy were the lab rats traveling in their time capsules and were the fore runners of people who today suffer heart conditions.

In the absence of the spectrum of minerals and vitamins which we need to maintain full good health, people become ill.

As a species, we are suffering a self-inflicted epidemic, or I should say, a series of self-inflicted epidemics simply because we don't get the right nutrients and/or anything like the correct amount or the needed amount of Vitamin C in our diets.

CHAPTER 3

SCURVY

Heart disease is a misnomer! The disease is characterised by scab-like build-ups that slowly grow on the walls of blood vessels. The underlying disease process reduces the supply of blood to the heart and other organs, resulting in angina, "heart cramp", heart attack and stroke. The correct terminology for this disease is "chronic scurvy", a subclinical form of the classic Vitamin C deficiency disease.

The findings of the Canadian team led by G.C. Willis MD were confirmed in the late 1980s by the world's then leading scientist, Linus Pauling PhD (1901 – 1994). Pauling, who was a double Nobel prize winner, alerted the world in lectures, in writings and on video after he and his associates conducted experiments that confirmed Dr. Willis' findings. To date this alert has never made its way into a mainstream media outlet and cardiologists are taught routinely to tell their patients that there is no connection between Vitamin C and heart disease.

From a scientific standpoint, if a medical doctor, or anyone, tries to challenge the true nature of cardiovascular disease, they must be able to cite experiments that refute the Pauling/Willis chronic scurvy hypothesis. Such experiments have never been published which is because they don't exist and have not been done!

The knowledge that heart disease is a form of scurvy has been suppressed from the time that the first series of Willis' articles were published in the Canadian Medical Association Journal in the early 1950s. Inexplicably since the 1950s, no article favourable to Vitamin C and its connection with atherosclerosis have appeared in reputable medical journals that are widely read by medical doctors.

The Linus Pauling video

In a 1992 lecture recorded on video, Dr. Linus Pauling explained the reason atherosclerosis forms on the walls of arteries when Vitamin C is deficient. He explained how a specific form of cholesterol causes plaques, compensating for low levels of Vitamin C, and why this discovery of a rapid cure for chronic scurvy includes the amino acid lysine.

There's no doubt that the news of this cure has been suppressed, otherwise most of the public would have learned that twice Nobel prize winner, Linus Pauling, has suggested it. In fact Linus Pauling made the claim of an outright cure for heart disease using Vitamin C at that time.

Because this cure cannot be patented and because Vitamin C is relatively cheap to produce, then the pharmaceutical industry has no interest in it whatever, nor do their dependants in the medical profession.

The greater majority of these people probably have no idea of the existence of this research and its findings which is deeply regrettable since this condition has cost many many lives.

Débâcle over cholesterol-lowering statin drugs

Following on in this vein, Cholesterol-lowering statin drugs have become the top selling class of prescription drugs with most people reaching middle age now being routinely put on these drugs as a preventive measure.

Vitamin C, which is a fraction of the price of statins, has the very same cholesterol-lowering property as the statin drugs and Vitamin C is a powerful anti-cholesterol agent. The Vitamin C molecule inhibits the same enzyme (HMG CoA reductase) that the cholesterol-lowering statin drugs inhibit and the big advantage is that it does so without depleting the body's supply of coenzyme Q10.

This blockage of coenzyme Q10 synthesis is a serious action for statin drugs that cause fatigue, muscle pain and skeletal myopathy (a grave deterioration of muscle). All advertisements in Canada must carry the coenzyme Q10 statin depletion warning, but this fact is not widely publicised elsewhere.

Transient global amnesia

Former NASA astronaut and USAF flight surgeon Duane Graveline MD believes that the statin drug lipitor caused his own case of transient global amnesia, a statin drug-associated memory dysfunction (and this happened whilst flying!). He's written a book, Statin Drugs; Side-Effects and the Misguided War on Cholesterol.

CHAPTER 4

FURTHER PROOF

Chronic scurvy verified by cardioretinometry and reversed with Vitamin C

It's long been known that human arteries weaken without Vitamin C and as a necessary nutritional support. Dr. Pauling and his associates theorised with Willis that such plaque formation will serve to strengthen weak arteries because they appear most often when the blood pressure is highest. This condition is most properly characterised as chronic scurvy.

Dr. Sydney Bush DOpt of the United Kingdom discovered that atheromas can be reversed in those patients instructed to take from 3,000 milligram to 10,000 milligram Vitamin C daily (the amount depending on the effect on the retinal arteries). Dr. Bush made this discovery while studying eye infections in contact lens wearers. Vitamin C was being tested as a preventative measure for these infections and serendipitously Dr. Bush noted that atheromas disappeared in the patients taking Vitamin C. He reported that some patients required as much as 10,000 milligram daily to reverse soft atheromas.

Dr. Bush has invented a new diagnostic technique which he calls cardio-retinometry and be believes that this method of diagnosis will revolutionise cardiology.

Dr. Bush has also promoted the idea that chronic scurvy not only exists but can be accurately measured. Eye doctors can now easily diagnose this condition by examining the microscopic arteries behind the eye before any symptoms of heart disease appear. Thanks to Dr. Bush, we now know that Vitamin C will reverse this condition in short order at the optimum dosage determined by cardioretinometry.

Reversing coronary heart disease

The atheroma of the retinal arteries is a virtually perfect surrogate outcome predictor of coronary heart disease and will continue to be so as long as the eyes are connected to the rest of the system. The modern electronic eye camera/microscopes with high definition magnification facility show the impacting of the cholesterol beautifully and also its re-dissolving into the bloodstream when the system is restored to balance. This is seen in arterioles, too small to be seen with the naked eye.

Dr. Bush now has evidence that even calcified "hard" plaques can be reversed over the course of two years on a high Vitamin C intake. This development throws a hammer into the government's recommended daily allowance of 60 milligram and the 2,000 milligram tolerable allowance. These are nonsense!

<u>Heal Yourself!</u>
A safe and effective answer to the most common form of heart disease – plaques forming over weak arteries – is 6,000 milligram to 18,000 milligram Vitamin C daily to strengthen the arteries. Dr. Pauling's invention of administering high dosed lysine, 2,000 milligram to 6,000 milligram, resolves existing plaques. This combination appears to work in most individuals within <u>ten days</u> with the correct dosage.

Congenital heart defects and heart damage

Harvard medical researchers found that Vitamin C was the only one of 880 substances tested that caused heart and muscles to regenerate from stem cells.

Heart Failure

Many people experience a remission of heart failure after they adopt Pauling's Vitamin C and lysine therapy. However, there is much evidence that the cause of heart failure in most people is the coenzyme Q10 deficiency. This vitamin-like coenzyme is required in our fuel cells, the mitochondria, in order to manufacture the body's fuel, adenosine triphosphate (ATP).

Several other vitamins are required for the human body to produce its own Co.Q10 and humans are known to synthesize less Co.Q10 as we age.

Pharmaceutical drugs and all the cholesterol lowering statin drugs block the body's production of Co.Q10. Therefore it can be accurately stated that these drugs cause a form of heart disease; heart failure.

High blood pressure/hypertension

Blood pressure normally elevates during times of stress for short periods. The higher blood pressure ensures that glucose and other nutrients enter the cells in order to aid response to the stress. It's also normal for high blood pressure to normalise after the stressful event passes.

According to discussions in the British Medical Journal, ophthalmologists have noticed that the plaques form in microscopic retinal arteries before the onset of elevated blood pressure. Pauling's therapy is an effective treatment for hypertension, as are other nutrients such as magnesium, B6 and the amino acid arginine. Health journalist, Bill Sardi, believes that 200 milligrams of Vitamin B6 is more effective than many prescription drugs for hypertension.

Calcified arteries and osteoporosis

Many heart patients have hard or calcified arteries. This makes heart attack more likely because blood vessels are unable to dilate properly in the event of a clot or blockage. The most probable cause of excess calcium building up in the arteries of the heart patients is the use of blood thinners. These prescription medications either simulate or block Vitamin K and they're routinely prescribed.

High dose Vitamin K reduces calcium in soft tissues and is considered a standard treatment for osteoporosis in Japan. The vitamin acts as a hormone and helps remove calcium from soft tissues into the bone.

Heart Attack

Strong Vitamin C/lysine fortified arteries are less likely to rupture. If there's no rupture, there will be no clot. If there's no clot, there will be no heart attack caused by a blockage of blood to the heart. World Health Organisation researchers have discovered that low serum Vitamin E is a 70% better predictor of heart attack than either hypertension (high blood pressure) or high cholesterol.

Also, K.K. Teo and others have discovered that a magnesium injection immediately after a heart attack saved 55% of those who would have died (British Medical Journal 303;1499-1503, 1991).

CHAPTER 5

THE BEGINNING OF LIFE ON EARTH.

Two billion years ago a species of cyanobacteria evolved which covered the earth and changed the atmosphere.

These cyanobacteria, which are a bit like the spirulina you can buy in health food stores today, release a lot of free oxygen. Back then this free oxygen killed all organisms except those that developed a mechanism to deal with oxygen poisoning.

Oxygen, although it's vital to life as we know it, is poisonous.

This is because the use of oxygen creates highly reactive toxic bi-products called superoxides or free radicals which can damage any part of the body, including the immune system.

These are destroyed, or I should say, "mopped-up" in the body by enzyme complexes called superoxide dismutase (SODS). Dr. Richard Cutler of the National Institute on Ageing has shown that the SOD level in primates is highly correlated with longevity.

Fortunately, we don't have to rely solely on SODS because during our evolution our bodies also developed mechanisms to use the nutrient anti-oxidants Vitamin C, E Selenium and turmeric as very effective free radical controllers.

These offer protection against levels of radiation that would otherwise kill us in about 72 hours!

Salts

Three billion years ago when the earth was still hot and covered by an atmosphere thick with dust and smoke, water formed in the atmosphere and rocks and it started to rain. Over millions of years the rain dissolved chemicals from the dust and gases in the atmosphere and since this rain was highly acidic, it also dissolved mineral salts and trace elements from the rocks and the soil.

Ultimately, these were transported down streams and rivers into the sea where they accumulated to form salt water. This salt water contained every mineral and trace element that was available in the earth's crust and atmosphere at that time and to this day the seas contain at least 85 different mineral salts and trace elements. These chemicals combined and recombined to form a vast array of chemical combinations, ultimately combining to form the basic building blocks of life on earth.

All of these are essential to life and we have recently established that every nutrient and essential element operates by multiple interactions in the human body.

Prior to the appearance of cyanobacteria and the oxygen they produced, the only way energy could be produced in the chemical soup of our seas was by fermentation. Slowly, as our early large-celled protein ancestors developed, there was very little energy available to them, particularly as they only had fermentation to draw on and were made of relatively large clumsy macromolecules in which the electrons were held firmly in their orbits and have no mobility.

Electrons are the small negatively-charged particles that surround the atomic core of a molecule. To have a flow of energy, these have to move from molecule to molecule. This is called electron transport.

The only electron conductor/acceptor available to early dark life was a weak chemical mixture called methyl-glyoxal. This couldn't conduct energy very well but when attached to the proteins, it was a start and dark life/fermentation quickly cashed in on this advantage by beginning to form proper cells with cell walls and nuclei.

This is essentially the first step on life's ladder and one which I shall return to in the next chapter on Vitamin C.

Blood

It will come as no surprise since we originated, as did all life, in the sea, to learn that our blood has more or less the same mineral profile that the sea had in the Cambrian era about 2 billion years ago. The same applies to all life which began in the sea.

This primeval sea is the perfect electrolyte, very able to transport electrons through the metabolic pathways of our body, and is the essential conductor of life.

Without salt in our diet we cannot live, since without it there can be no intercellular communication and our bodies begin to fall apart.

Just make sure it's sea salt or ancient rock salt that you are consuming (you'll see why on page 53).

Chapter 6

VITAMIN C

Vitamin C is essential to life and is the mechanism by which life was able to use oxygen and thereby to vigorously proliferate.

Vitamin C or L-ascorbic acid, is a rather simple substance, its chemical formula being $C_6H_8O_6$. It's closely related to carbohydrates; indeed in the cells of plants and most animals (with man being one of the exceptions) it's made from the simple sugar glucose (dextrose, grape sugar, corn sugar), which has the formula $C_6H_{12}O_6$ (not a lot of difference). Ascorbic acid is a weak acid with an acidic strength between that as citric acid (the principle acid in citrus fruits) and acetic acid, the acid of vinegar. More importantly, it's also a chemical-reducing agent capable of combining with oxygen and serving as an anti-oxidant. As an anti-oxidant it's effective, together with Vitamin E, in protecting cell membranes against damage by oxidation. In addition to this function and its function in the synthesis of collagen, it's involved in a host of other bio-chemical processes in the human body.

The Energy Bridge

Vitamin C is essential to the mechanism of life because it can easily pass one of its electrons to oxygen. When it does this, its remaining structure becomes destabilised and is known as a very reactive free radical. This is a molecule that's lost an electron and needs to absorb another as quickly as possible to get back into balance. It does this by taking an electron from the methylglyoxal attached to the protein. (You remember I mentioned methylglyoxal as a very early mechanism of electron transport which developed shortly after life got started on this planet). By taking an electron from methylglyoxal, this enables the protein to pass more electrons down this chain to the oxygen. This gives rise to a much higher level of electronic activity than could otherwise take place.

Electron transport

This bridge from the protein to the methylglyoxal to the Vitamin C to oxygen, is basic to most life on this planet, and acts both as a bridge and an essential buffer. The reason for this is that if oxygen could take electrons straight from protein, we'd burn up in rapid oxidation. As it is, it's a regulated process requiring lots of Vitamin C.

In this pivotal role, Vitamin C is different from all of the other vitamins and since we don't get nearly enough in our food, it's essential that you take a Vitamin C supplement. Everybody's metabolism is different to the extent that some of us appear to be almost different species from others (this is not the case) having different digestive systems and different internal layout. However, the minimum intake of Vitamin C to remain fully healthy and to have one's blood fully oxygenated is 3,000 milligram a day and for other individuals it's 10,000 milligram a day. This can only be established by trial and error (or blood tests) but is vital to both the immune system and to longevity.

Essential Fuel for your immune system
Concerning the immune system, T-lymphocyte cells are our main mechanism of cellular immunity. Keeping the T-cells in top condition is critical to the prevention of ageing. They protect the body against foreign cells, bacteria, fungus, virus and allergens and they also help the body resist cancer

and auto-immune diseases. Defective T-cell function accompanies most degenerative diseases including cancer, rheumatoid arthritis, multiple sclerosis, diabetes mellitus and ulcerative colitis.

A big part of the ageing process is the gradual decline in T-cells which occurs even without any apparent disease. T-cells have a very high level of Vitamin C but with age degeneration the level drops progressively and we lose our resistance to disease. The Vitamin C level of T-cells and companion white cells, is essential in fighting disease because if you do get a virus or other infection, it drops very quickly.

The more severe the infection the worse the loss, unless you take a C supplement. Dietary Vitamin C reduces the loss of Vitamin C in the T-cells and can considerably reduce symptoms.

Moreover concerning the use of oxygen, blood volume and red blood cell counts vary with exercise and with the help of Vitamin C, new capillaries grow in the heart and skeletal muscles to carry the improved blood supply.

Accordingly, there's a huge improvement in performance since the Vitamin C helps balance the pH of the blood which is then made more alkaline. An alkaline bloodstream is capable of carrying considerably more oxygen than an acidic one and I'll deal with this later when I come on to alkalinity.

About Vitamin C intake

Vitamin C cannot be stored in the body, it's got to be replenished regularly. However, the blood will only absorb so much Vitamin C regardless of how much you may take at one time. For example, I take between 5 and 10 grams a day and how much is excreted will depend on my body's specific need at that time.

When I'm under stress I need more Vitamin C and at other times perhaps less. This intake will rapidly cause deep saturation and then will taper off gradually returning to the previous level, so that since Vitamin C is inexpensive, it's better to waste a bit than to take too little. Vitamin C has proved beyond any doubt to be totally non-toxic and since its discovery by Albert Szent-Györgyi, abundant research has proved its efficacy.

In 1970 after the publication of Linus Pauling's book on the treatment of the common cold, Vitamin C became a temporary fad, but when Linus Pauling (two-time Nobel prize winner) and Dr. Ewen Cameron published their three studies on the importance of Vitamin C in cancer treatment, it has been roundly attacked and many attempts have been made to discredit its usefulness by a pharmaceutical industry which cannot patent it and therefore cannot profit from it.

The animal kingdom

Because of a 60 million year old genetic defect, humans have been deprived of the ability to make their own ascorbate in their livers. Plants manufacture their own Vitamin C with great efficiency. Animals are also able to make their own Vitamin C, with three great exceptions:-

The fruit bat, the guinea pig, and the primates; (monkeys, apes and you and I!)

It seems ironic that a goat, which is similar in weight to a man, can manufacture 13 grams of Vitamin C daily (and double, even quadruple that amount under stress) and yet you and I are left dependent upon food for our Vitamin C supply. Unwittingly nature dealt us a grievous blow.

How did this happen?
I believe that our distant ancestors were living in areas with a plentiful supply of fruit. They could eat so much fruit at that time that nature decided they got all the Vitamin C they needed in their diets. Because there seemed to be no point in the body's manufacturing Vitamin C this ability was lost since it makes no sense to nature to carry around the hardware for providing the enzyme L-gulonolactone oxidase if it's not needed.

Unfortunately, from a biological standpoint, we no longer live in a jungle where we can walk up and pick a piece of Vitamin C rich fruit whenever we feel hungry. This is a tragic turning point in our development, made worse by the fact that it's left us with an inborn desire for sweets, which was put there by nature to make sure we ate fruit that was ripe (and took in a good supply of Vitamin C).

Our bio-chemistry is the loser. We fail to get the massive amounts of Vitamin C nature intended us to have and we get fat through eating too many sweet things.

Vitamin C – an essential food

Mankind can't get enough Vitamin C from his ordinary diet and not even from a very fruit-rich diet. The reason for this lies in the physiological difference between animals and plants. There is a difference here between animals and humans, insofar as animals manufacture large amounts of collagen which is their principle micro-molecule (in place of the cellulose manufactured by plants), and ascorbic acid is required for the synthesis of collagen.

Therefore animals need ascorbic acid in greater supply than plants do as one of the basic building blocks of their bodies. Accordingly, any animal strain which lacks the ability to synthesise ascorbic acid would probably die out very rapidly as the supply of the plant-food diet would not fulfil its needs. Since animals can manufacture Vitamin C in their bodies, they are able to apply this to the manufacture of collagen, whereas we humans cannot. Accordingly, we have to get it from our diet and by checking the amounts of several Vitamins present in 110 raw, natural plant foods, the amounts of vitamins corresponding to one day's food for an adult turn out to be (for several vitamins) about three times the usual dietary intake!

But for Vitamin C the amount in plant foods is 2,300 milligram, which is 51 times the average intake in an ordinary diet. This indicates very strongly that we all ought to be vegetarians but also there's something very special about Vitamin C.

The average amount of Vitamin C in a day's ration of 8 foods with the highest content is 12,000 milligram and our early ancestor who lost the ability to synthesise ascorbic acid was probably living in a tropical valley where these and similar high C foods provided this large amount of the vitamin.

The other primates have, for the most part, continued to live in tropical areas where the food has a high concentration of Vitamin C, but human beings have spread into other areas and their intake of Vitamin C has decreased to such an extent as to cause the health of nearly every person to suffer.

Hypoascorbemia

We also suffer from hypoascorbemia, a deficiency of ascorbate in the blood, or in other words the lack of Vitamin C. Accordingly, when we spread out from the jungles of Africa a couple of hundred thousand years ago, we passed the pivot point or turning point where we became shorter-lived and congenitally less healthy because our external supply of Vitamin C was dramatically reduced. Human beings with a high intake of Vitamin C manufacture more antibody molecules than those with a lower intake and antibodies or anti-toxins are protein molecules that have the power of recognising "not self" cells and combining with them, thus helping to mark them for destruction by the body's normal processes.

Self and not self

There is another complex of protein molecules called complement that is involved in an essential way in the process of destruction of foreign cells and malignant cells. It's been shown that an increased intake of Vitamin C significantly increases the amount of the first component of complement C1 esterase, without which the whole complement cascade is inoperable and the "not self" cells could not be destroyed. That Vitamin C is required in man for the synthesis of C1 esterase is proved by the fact that the component of complement contains protein molecules that are similar to the molecules of collagen which are known to require Vitamin C for their synthesis.

Albeit on leaving the jungles our diet dramatically reduced in Vitamin C, yet the diet of Palaeolithic man was known by research to have contained 83% of green stuff, i.e. enzyme and Vitamin C rich fresh food (whereas modern diets are enzyme poor because of cooking and preservatives, are certainly not fresh and have very little Vitamin C in them).

CHAPTER 7

IODINE.

Iodine is a vital antioxidant in life's processes. It protects against free radicals (superoxide anion, hydrogen peroxide and hydroxyl radical that oxygen breeds). Iodine increases the antioxidant status of human serum similar to but on a different vector from Vitamin C.

Iodine induces programmed cell death. This process is essential to growth and development and is also vital for destroying cells that represent a threat to the integrity of the organism (like cancer cells).

Fibrocystic Breast Disease
Russian researchers first showed in 1966 that iodine effectively relieves signs and symptoms of fibrocystic breast disease and in 1993 a Canadian study published in the Canadian Journal of Surgery, likewise found that iodine relieves signs and symptoms of fibrocystic breast disease in 70% of their patients.

The FDA regard iodine as a natural substance not a drug and most physicians and surgeons view iodine from a narrow perspective as an antiseptic that disinfects drinking water and prevents surgical wounds' infection. It's also needed by the thyroid to make thyroid hormones.

The thyroid gland needs iodine to synthesise hormones that regulate metabolism and steer growth and development and whilst the thyroid only needs trace elements of iodine, there's a vast body of evidence that a higher dose of iodine will prevent a whole spectrum of disorders. The Nobel Laureate Dr. Albert Szent-Györgyi (1893 to 1986), the physician who discovered Vitamin C, widely recommended iodine's use as a sort of universal medicine.

<u>Seaweed</u>

To maintain whole body sufficiency of iodine requires 12.5 milligram a day. This is similar to what the Japanese consume with the seaweed in their diet. The vast majority of people retain a substantial amount of this dosage and many require 50 milligrams a day for several months before they excrete 90% of it, indicating that their body has reached its equilibrium. In fact the body will hold 1,500 milligram with only 3% of that being held in the thyroid gland. Thyroid function remains unchanged using this amount of iodine and since it removes toxic halogens, fluoride and bromide from the body, we should all take at least 2 drops of Lugol's solution or 1 iodoral tablet a day.

Until recently the chief source of iodine in the western diet was table salt. However, the bulk of people now buy salt without iodine which is called table salt but has all the trace elements driven off. Accordingly, over the last three decades people who used to use iodised table salt have now unwittingly decreased their consumption by 65%. Moreover, high concentrations of chloride in manufactured salt inhibit absorption of its sister halogen iodine.

A Crucial Nutrient
The intestines only absorb 10% of the iodine present in iodised table salt, so in order to stay healthy it's vital to increase one's intake of iodine. You will find that everything in your body functions better (even your brain) once it's nourished by the iodine it needs. The key here is to think of iodine not as a remedy but as a nutrient that's crucial to all aspects of health and can help enormously in recovery from cancer.

Your doctor will probably say that you get all the iodine you need from fish and if you could consume 20 lbs of fish a day and withstand the mercury, PCPs and etc. now present in all fish you probably could! However, 2 drops of Lugol's per day in a glass of water is safe and an extremely conservative dose and you might like to take more to help yourself recover.

Iodine supplement brings about an immediate lifting of spirits in mildly depressed people and does wonders to alleviate crankiness. It also helps banish long-established migraines!

Radiation poisoning
Finally, because iodine in the cells prevents the uptake of radioactive iodine (a different substance) then iodine is extremely effective in preventing you from suffering from mild radiation poisoning which we're all susceptible to with the increase in background radiation caused by atomic testing and atomic reactor disasters.

Our current exposure to toxicalytes, fluoride, bromide, tetrachlorates and isocyanate is higher than humans have ever been exposed to in the past. Fluoride, a strong neuro-toxin, is added to drinking water, allegedly to stop tooth decay, and we also ingest fluoride from sources such as pesticides, medicines, food, salt, toothpaste and health supplements.

Similarly, bromide is another toxic halide which is everywhere. It's got an antibacterial function similar to chlorine and is used as a fumigant for agriculture and termites. It's a virulent pesticide that kills insects on contact and when it's injected into the soil everything dies.

Cheap & Nasty
Bromide is cheap and abundant and appears in a vast number of food stuffs and has replaced iodine as a dough conditioner for bread and is used widely in the milk industry because of its effective bactericide properties.

This is where iodine comes in. It helps the body eliminate fluoride, bromide, lead, calcium, arsenic, aluminium and mercury, and since it's now been replaced by bromine in bread and milk, there's no longer a way to eliminate the bromine.

Morbid Obesity

The ubiquitous nature of bromide in food stuffs, particularly sodas, gives rise to morbid obesity. When oil is placed in a bowl and bromine is stirred in, the bromine will slowly turn the liquid oil into a solid until it becomes so stiff that the spoon won't move. This happens in your body and goes a long way toward explaining the cause of our epidemic of obesity. Years of drinking sodas that are loaded with brominated vegetable oil solidifies body fat.

To conclude, adequate iodine levels are necessary for proper immune system function. About 1.5 billion people around the world live in areas of iodine deficiency and iodine is responsible for the production of all the hormones of the body and 20% of the body's store of iodine is in the skin. Accordingly, if you want to recover your health as quickly as possible, it is vital that you begin to use iodine as part of your diet.

CHAPTER 8

WATER

One of the reasons you got heart problems in the first place is that you've been seriously dehydrated for most of your life. Chronic dehydration is the root cause of many diseases that we confront in society today and once you take this on board and start drinking at least 3 pints of water spread out through the day, your overall health will improve significantly.

Our bodies evolved in the sea and the role of water in the bodies of all living species (mankind included) hasn't changed since the first creation of life in salt water. When we evolved into amphibians, living in fresh water and then on the land, we had to develop a body-water-preservation system in order to carry our environment with us.

The human body is composed of 25% solid matter and 75% water (the brain tissue consisting of 85% water). And it's assumed by science that the solutes (the solids that are dissolved in or carried in the blood serum of the body) regulate the activity of the body. In fact, without adequate supplies of water, the spectrum of reactions which support life in the body simply cannot function adequately. In order to maintain an adequate supply of water to the vital organs, various peripheral systems are shut down as the vital organs take priority. The brain, for example, whilst it's $1/50^{th}$ of the total body weight, receives 18 to 20% of blood circulation and when it doesn't get this, various short-term non-essential systems are shut down reducing enzymic activity and storing up problems which later manifest as a whole variety of diseases.

The Cholesterol Myth

In regard to heart disease, high blood cholesterol is a sign that the cells of the body are employing a defence mechanism against the osmotic force of the blood that keeps drawing water out through the cell membranes, or that the concentrated blood cannot release sufficient water to go through the cell membrane and maintain normal cell functions.

Cholesterol is a natural binder, which when poured in the gaps of the cell membrane, makes the cell wall impervious to the passage of water. The manufacture of cholesterol is part of the natural design for the protection of living cells against dehydration. In living cells that possess a nucleus, cholesterol is the agent that regulates the amount of water that will pass the cell membrane and in living cells that do not possess a nucleus, the make-up of fatty acids employed in the manufacture of cell membranes gives it the power to survive dehydration and drought.

Cholesterol production in the cell membrane is part of the cell's survival system. It's a necessary substance. Its success denotes dehydration.

If you provide an adequate supply of water to your body (i.e. three pints a day spread out through the day) then in a relatively short space of time, your cholesterol levels will decrease and you will feel a lot better.

Chapter 9

OBESITY

Years of dehydration, and years of ill-advised diet have caused your body to accumulate a host of toxins in its structure. This is largely because of one of the body's cleverest priorities is to maintain the pH level of your blood at around 7.2, that is to say, slightly alkaline.

This alkalinity is necessary because a more alkaline bloodstream can carry more dissolved oxygen than can an acidic one. The body's main priority here, being to supply an adequate flow of electrons via the oxygen, via the bloodstream to all the organs of the body.

In order to maintain this beneficial alkaline quotient in the blood, your body shunts acidic toxins into its "storage areas". This is why fatty acids form as accumulated fat in those areas of the body such as the buttocks, upper thighs, back of the arms and so forth where obesity begins. Toxic fats and fats containing the whole range of toxic-food additives that are lavished on our food these days, accumulate in these back waters as part of a process designed to keep our bloodstreams healthy.

As you begin to take enhanced levels of Vitamin C, enhanced levels of iodine and enhanced levels of water, these fatty acids will begin to precipitate back into your bloodstream whence they will be removed by your liver and kidneys. This process of detoxification works much better and more quickly if you begin to take quantities of natural charcoal.

Charcoal
Natural charcoal (not activated) has two major functions to play in good health. The first is that it adsorbs over 4,000 known toxins (and quite probably a great many more that have been invented in the last century as food additives). By adsorbing these acidic toxins and taking them out of the system naturally, natural charcoal supplements and supports the activity of your liver and kidneys helping to rapidly clear up your bloodstream. This helps the bloodstream to return to its natural alkalinity within a reasonably short space of time.

Natural charcoal has been used for thousands of years by our species (and many others) and is chemically inert, therefore completely harmless and can be taken with impunity and with very good effect over a period of many years.

C_{60} adds energy

The second function of charcoal and one which derives from its high content of the molecule C_{60} (the basic molecule of all life on earth) is the fact that it transports into the body a cloud of electrons which adds significantly to the body's energy levels. These electrons seek out damaging free radicals and direct them down the metabolic pathways in the body, thereby preventing them from doing further damage.

So in this way the charcoal, which I'm recommending, helps purge your body of toxins, helps re-energise your body and helps to protect it against oxidative damage. A triple whammy well worth employing.

Chapter 10

CHARCOAL

Everything alive on earth today is, as far as we know, carbon based. Until recently it was thought there were only three basic types of carbon available on earth and none of those were capable of providing a structure on which life could evolve. Graphite is too malleable – diamond is too rigid and far too hard and soot is formless. So the type of carbon upon which life was based was until recently a mystery. However, in 1985 carbon C_{60} was discovered and this is now called fullerene after Buckminster Fuller, the famous architect. (C_{60} has a geodesic structure like the geodesic dome invented by Buckminster Fuller.)

C_{60} is hollow like a ball and only three angstroms across, just enough space to enclose one other atom in its structure.   So C_{60} which is pure carbon has a form of structure which is strong, resilient and biologically active. It can combine with other elements.

Adsorption

C_{60} active or potentised charcoal has a unique ability to adsorb toxins. This adsorption process causes atoms or molecules of a substance to form on or bind to its surface.

Tiny particles of charcoal are riddled with a network of crevices, cracks and tunnels such that the combined surface area of a one centimetre cube would unfold to a 1,000 square centimetres. This tremendous surface area is capable of adsorbing well over 4,000 acidic substances by physically binding molecules to the charcoal in a process known as van der Waal forces.

Rogue Oxygen Species

Van der Waal forces are electromagnetic in nature and there is a vast body of scientific evidence showing that C_{60} charcoal not only adsorbs over 4,000 different toxic substances, but also carries (owing to its electron cloud) a substantial burst of energy into the body where it is used to capture and transmit free radicals (excess electrons left over from an oxidative burst) guiding these down the metabolic pathways of the body.

Charcoal derived carbon C_{60} is used by the body to build a healthy carbon network which forms all important pathways along which oxygen moves. In its absence, oxygen burned in the cells as fuel forms free radicals which are an oxygen species which can do great harm, but when oxygen is "burned" by the cells in the presence of C_{60}, this forms a spherical cage around the rogue oxygen species and reinstalls them in their proper respiratory pathways. Effectively this activity acts also as an antiviral, antifungal and antibacterial mechanism. It doesn't kill these three, but simply deactivates them by temporarily neutralising their positively charged nucleic acids - i.e. they are less of a threat whilst in the presence of C_{60}-rich charcoal molecules.

Finally, C_{60} charcoal has an affinity for acidic toxins adsorbing over 4,000 known elements of these species. By adsorbing acidic toxins from the gut and bloodstream and indeed from the entire system, this helps to rebalance the pH in the body helping it to become more alkaline, and therefore better oxygenated. In this role charcoal C_{60} performs a vital function in the recovery of cells' energy levels helping to switch them back from cancer (the dark state of life) into normal healthy cells driven by the citrate cycle – light life.

Rheology = Functional Shape

The C_{60} molecule prevents free radical damage by forming a spherical cage around them (i.e. the free radicals) and reinstalling them in their proper respiratory pathways. It also revitalises the health of cells which are "run down" and losing their shape. This is a vital function in that it restores their ability to carry oxygen! Ergo, it provides a reliable and stable template for cellular rheology. This is a critical step in the process of reviving cancerous cells and turning them back into normal body cells.

If you take 2 - 4 x 250mg natural charcoal capsules every night with a glass of water, not only will your entire system become a lot more healthy, courtesy of the detox, but the energy that this wonderful substance transmits throughout the body will help your cells recover their true identity.

At this point in this book I stop writing specifically about how you can quite easily recover from so called "Heart Disease", and go on to write about how to slow down the ageing process.

In fact, the two subjects are interlinked so one bears on the other; but in the case of the anti-ageing strategies, I am more concerned to deal with the electro-magnetic aspects of our lives and how you can improve / enhance them to benefit you.

Chapter 11

HOW TO SLOW THE AGEING PROCESS

MAGNETISM AND EARTHING

The human body is made up of up to 90% water. This water has a high saline content which makes it a very good conductor of electricity and the cerebro-spinal fluid is made up of almost pure Vitamin C which is an extraordinarily good conductor of electrons. Finally, the brain is made up of totally unsaturated fatty proteins so that it behaves as an organic, body-temperature super conductor. There being no resistance to the passage of electromagnetic currents through its medium.

The whole structure of our bodies, and particularly the brain-spine complex, act as a perfect biological antenna conducting fluctuations in the earth's electromagnetic field throughout the entire structure. These fluctuations have a major effect on our hormones and as far back as 1964, L. Gross showed that a small difference in a magnetic field can produce physical effects:-

Magnetic fields modify the wave functions of electrons in macro-molecules, producing a greater paramagnetic susceptibility, which leads to a slow-down in reaction speed and the rate at which the RNA and DNA are synthesised.

In other words, the replication of DNA macro-molecules is mediated by the action of the fluctuation in the earth's magnetic field. DNA is very sensitive to magnetic fields and turns perpendicularly to a magnetic field.
Its electromagnetic sympathy is implicit in its structure and behaviour since it's a left-handed spiral form.

The earth's magnetic field has fluctuated over the millennia and these fluctuations have had a profound effect on humankind, particularly on our life span.

Dr. Okai of Kyorin University in Japan has discovered an increase in the life span of red blood cells in the bodies of mice and a strong magnetic field environment. Human beings are not mice but our metabolisms are very similar and Dr. Okai hypothesises that the substantial increase in longevity in his test subjects may be due to the sterilising action and other positive life prolonging attributes possessed by the magnetic field.

Magnetic fields on health

Any conducting substance moving in the presence of a magnetic field generates electricity. Accordingly, the blood flow generates electricity which ionises the blood and as we're seeing when any molecule is ionised, it's very active. Accordingly, the magnetic field and your heart pumping energy force the separation of plus and minus ions, and these active ions have been detected to loosen and chip away plaque and cholesterol build up in the arteries.

In its active stage, each ion has an electric field which induces water to be hexagonally structured and active. Consequently, the water content of the blood is extremely sensitive to fluctuations in the earth's magnetic field and throughout the billions of years of our evolution, it's axiomatic that our life expectancy has fluctuated in direct proportion to the strength of the earth's magnetic field.

The decline of the field

The earth's magnetic field has been measurably declining for the last 300 years and it is postulated by many leading scientists that we are now entering a period of time when the earth's polarity will reverse. This has happened many times throughout history and is usually a time of much chaos, strife, ill-health and systemic collapse.

At this point, it's worth the mention that on a personal level, you can strengthen your own exposure to the earth's magnetic field by wearing a small array of magnets.

These significantly improve your circulation and the quality of your blood in ionic terms as well as boosting the hormonal activity within your structure.

The wearing of a properly constructed magnetic device actually strengthens the electrical currents in your body. This is because any electrolyte (such as human blood) moving through a magnetic field will have a strengthened electrical potential.

By properly constructed, I mean that the device must be negative toward the body and positive away, since the flow of magnetic gauss is from positive to negative. In this way we put energy into the flow rather than taking it out.

Diurnal flow

As it circles the earth the moon "pumps" the ionosphere up and down as it pulls the tides around the planet. This has the effect of pumping the energy flow of electrons from the negative earth to the positive ionosphere and this pumping action causes the electrons to flow along the metabolic pathways of the body which are the energy lines of classical acupuncture.

Using an electron microscope, one can actually see electrons entering and exiting the skin at acupuncture points where they form a helical flow which helix or vortex directs the pressure of the electronic flow in and out of the body. This is known in Chinese medicine as the flow of "chi" or "prana" in the Hindu tradition. Human beings, and indeed all living creatures, are subjected to this energy flow and have a magnetic sensitivity which in man is centred on the pineal gland (the third eye) which sensitivity in large part affects the electromagnetic activity in their bodies. By insulating oneself from this flow of energy, one is shortening one's life and damaging one's health.

Our new electronic environment

We depend on electricity for almost everything. We live in a world which is increasingly run and organised through electricity. This has given rise to a multitude of electrical machines which have become part of the fabric of our daily lives. The use of computers, televisions, central heating pumps, fluorescent lights, photocopiers, washing machines, radios and bedside lamps, plus a host of other equipment, have created a huge web of electrical wiring in every house, factory, public building and office. This complex new environment can have serious effects on our general health and well-being.

This is because the method of power generation, used in almost every electrical device or system in use on the planet today, is creating artificial spiral vortex fields at right angles to the current flow which rotate in the opposite direction to the ones which occur naturally and are used within living systems.

Boyers Binding Mechanism

In the human system, rhythmic patterns of activity throughout the organism are of a left-handed nature, they are the result of the movement of force fields which initially organised amino acid/matter into left-handed structures. These left-handed forces, the product of a natural magnetic field, continue to operate in a healthy body. When they are subjected to interference from fields rotating in the opposite direction, a break down in the signals can occur. Aberrant signals emanating from an oscillator in a disturbed pattern can bring about profoundly different growth instructions in single cells and this is nowadays a major stressor which can lead to cancerous states in the body. This is because the cells are receiving the wrong growth instructions from the DNA (which in normal function has a left-hand rotation) which is being stimulated by the wrong signals.

How to protect yourself

It is vital to good health and particularly to longevity to learn now how to protect yourself against the modern mechanically driven electromagnetic environment.

The planet is a 6 sextillion metric ton battery that is constantly being replenished by solar radiation, lightning and heat from its molten core. The rhythmic pulsations of natural energy flowing through and from the surface of the earth to the protective shields of the Van Allen belt, keep the biological machinery of life on earth running in rhythm and balance.

Each living creature is a collection of dynamic electrical circuits and in the complexity of our bodies, trillions of cells constantly transmit and receive energy in the course of their programmed bio-chemical reactions.

Our hearts, brains, nervous systems, muscles and immune systems are prime examples of electrical systems operating within our bio-electrical body. In a study published in 2005 by electrical engineer Roger Applewhite, two significant factors were confirmed:-

1. Electrons move from the body to the earth and vice-versa when the body is grounded. The effect is sufficient to maintain the body at the same negative-charged potential as the earth.

2. Grounding dramatically reduces the impact of electromagnetic fields on the body.

The Applewhite study showed the protective effect of earthing against environmental electric fields and in his classic lectures on physics in the early 1960s, Nobel Prize physicist, Richard Feynman describes the earth's subtle energies. The surface, as we have seen, has an abundance of electrons which give it a negative charge. If you're standing outside on a clear day wearing shoes or standing on an insulating surface, there is an electrical charge of some 350 volts between the earth and the top of your head if you're about 6 feet tall. That is to say, zero at ground level and 350 volts in the area of your head.

You don't get a shock because air is a relatively poor conductor and has virtually no electrical current flow.

If, on the other hand, you're standing outside in your bare feet, you are earthed, your whole body is in electrical contact with the earth's surface.

The Umbrella Effect

Your body is a relatively good conductor. Your skin and the earth's surface make a continuous charged surface at the same electrical potential. Therefore, any object in direct contact with the earth essentially becomes part of the earth and resides within the protective umbrella of the earth's natural electric field.

Accordingly, if you want to protect yourself from the worst effects of the modern mechanically driven electromagnetic environment, then it is important for you to walk barefoot on the earth for at least half an hour each day.

Earthing is dose related

The longer you are able to ground yourself in your daily life, the more stable, energetic and robust your body functions will be and the greater your ability to heal. The reason for this is that the human immune system evolved over millions of years. During this great span of time, we lived mostly in barefoot contact with the earth. We were naturally earthed. This meant that the biological clock of the body was continually calibrated by the pulse of the earth that governs the circadian rhythms of all life on the planet.

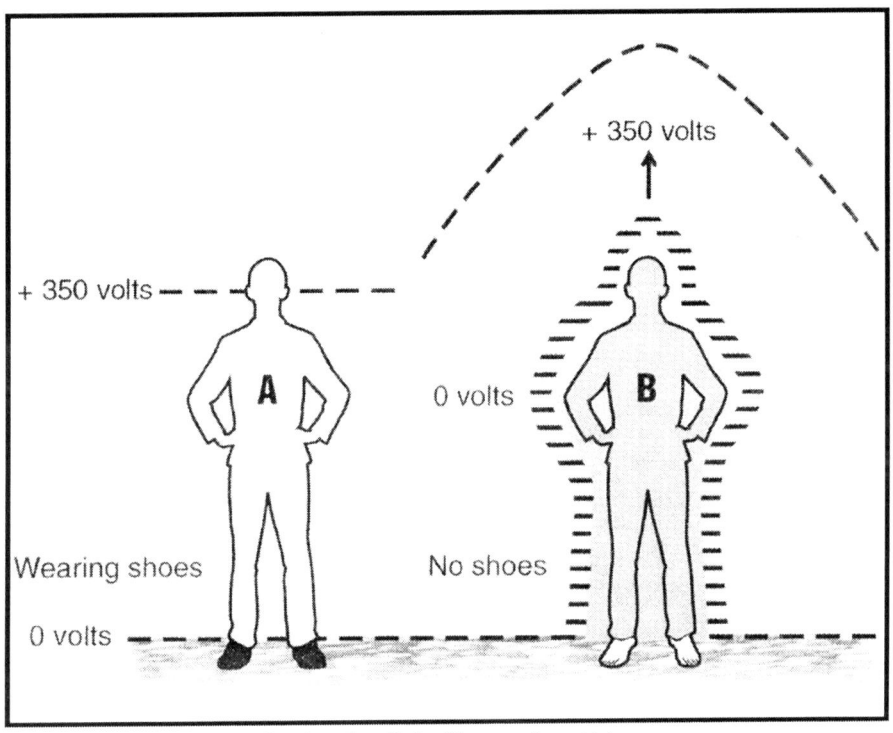

The 'umbrella' effects of earthing

Chapter 12

MOCCASINS AND MAGNETS

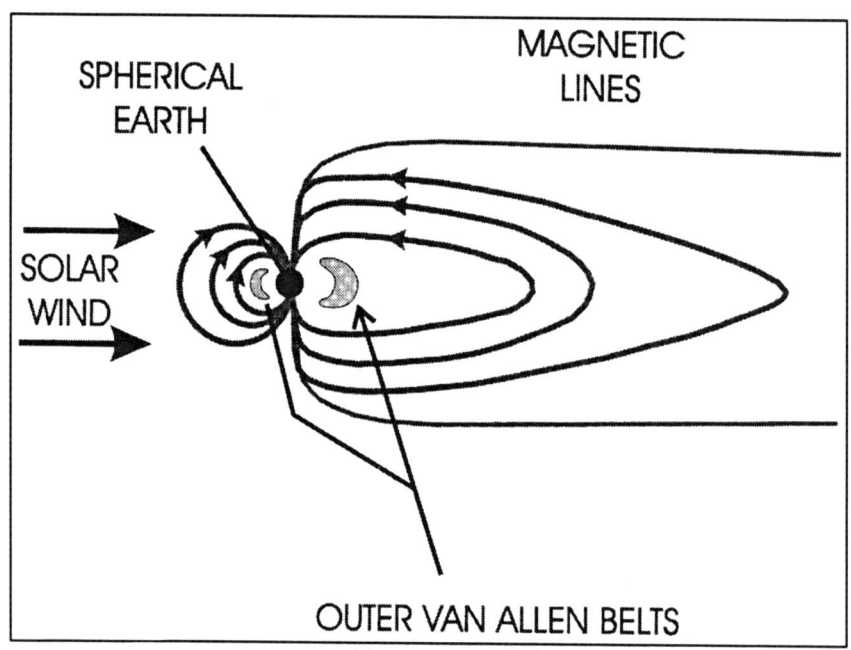

Earth's magnetic field

Disconnecting

What happens to the human body when it's separated from the subtle evolutionary signals from the earth was dramatically shown by experiments in Germany at the world famous Max Planck Institute during the 60s and 70s.

Researchers intentionally isolated volunteers for months at a time in underground rooms electrically shielded from the rhythms in the earth's electrical field. Patterns of body temperature, sleep, urinary excretion and other physiological activities were carefully monitored. All the participants developed a variety of abnormal or chaotic patterns. They experienced disturbed sleep and waking patterns, out of sync hormonal production and overall disruption in basic body regulation. Whilst we don't live underground, as did these volunteers, we live above the ground and on the ground but we've disconnected ourselves from these bio-rhythms by wearing shoes.

Natural Gait

The late Dr. William Rossi, a Massachusetts podiatrist and footwear industry historian, wrote in a 1999 article in Podiatry Management: "A natural gait is biomechanically impossible for any shoe wearing person, it took 4 million years to develop our unique human foot and our consequent distinctive form of gait – a remarkable feat of bio-engineering. Yet in only a thousand years and with one carelessly designed instrument, our shoes, we've warped the pure anatomical form of human gait, obstructing its engineering efficiency, afflicting it with strains and stresses and denying its natural grace of form and ease of movement head to foot".

He further wrote in Footwear News in 1997: "The Sole (or Plantar Surface of the Foot) is richly covered with some 1,300 nerve endings per square inch. That's more than found on any other part of the body of comparable size and is there to keep us in touch with the earth - the real physical world around us".

The paws of all animals are equally rich in nerve endings and the earth is covered with an electromagnetic layer from which every living thing including human beings draws energy.

The energy residing on the surface of the earth is primarily electrical and the central theme of this part of this paper is that we draw electrical energy through our feet in the form of free electrons fluctuating at many frequencies. These frequencies reset our biological clock and provide the body with electrical energy. The electrons themselves flow into the body, equalising and maintaining it at the electrical potential of the earth.

Moccasins

The original light weight soft sole, heelless and simple moccasin – a piece of crudely tanned leather that envelopes the foot and is fastened on with rawhide thongs – is possibly the closest we've ever come to an ideal shoe. It dates back more than 14,000 years.

To substantiate this, Dr. Morris Ghaly measured the circadian secretion of cortisol on people before and after they slept grounded over a period of a few weeks. The study was published in a 2004 issue of the Journal of Alternative and Complementary Medicine and the conclusion was:-

"Earthing during sleep resynchronises cortisol secretion more in alignment with its natural, normal rhythm – highest at 8am and lowest at midnight".

Whether you sleep grounded or walk barefoot on the earth, the effect of earthing out all of the unnatural energies impacting your body's antenna is profoundly beneficial.

Blood Thinning

Experiments conducted by Stephen Sinatra MD with a group of clinical physicians, PhD's working in the medical field, nurses and the author Clint Oba showed an astonishing effect on blood viscosity of grounding.

This experiment involved taking a drop of blood before and after 40 minutes of grounding by electro patches, and then examining the fresh unstained blood under a dark field microscope.

The after-grounding picture showed that people's blood dramatically changes within a short period of time after an individual is in contact with the earth. Specifically, there were considerably fewer formations of red blood cells associated with clamping and clotting. The blood appeared to be thinner.

The result suggested that individuals with heart disease and inflammatory thick blood (typical in cardiovascular disease and diabetes) may reap huge benefits from simply earthing themselves on a regular basis.

Inflammation and ageing

Inflammation comes in two forms, acute or chronic. The acute form takes place as an initial response to the body to harmful stimuli. It involves the mobilisation of plasma from the blood into the injured tissue and in the short-term this is a beneficial reaction.

On the other hand, chronic inflammation means a progressive shift in the type of activity going on at the site of the inflammation.

This occurs when you get simultaneous destruction and healing of the tissue, but also a harmful free-radical encroachment into healthy surrounding territory.

(Free radicals are the basis of chronic disease and the ageing process, particularly accelerated ageing and limited lifespan.)

<u>Pain</u>
This occurs when normal inflammation veers out of control because of the lost contact with the earth. People are suffering from an electron deficiency, that is to say not enough free electrons on hand to neutralise the rampaging free-radicals. Unfortunately, these go on to attack the adjacent healthy tissue in an ever expanding vicious cycle. The non-stop attack mode generates an auto-immune response manifesting as chronic inflammation and the immune system has run amuck. The pain generated in this process is entirely due to the positive free radical reactions and can be considerably assuaged by continually earthing the system/body on a regular basis.

<u>Jet Lag</u>
Earthing then considerably benefits each and every one of us, reduces chronic pain, energises us, reduces or eliminates jet lag, dramatically speeds healing and helps prevent bed sores, lessens hormonal and menstrual

problems, accelerates recovery from intense athletic activity, thins blood and improves blood pressure and flow. It normalises the body's biological rhythms, lowers stress and promotes calmness in the body by cooling down the nervous system and stress hormones. It improves sleep and protects the body against potentially health disturbing environmental electromagnetic forces.

To conclude, the wearing of magnetic bracelets and similar devices is highly beneficial as we have seen, as is the practice of earthing on a daily basis. It's now possible to buy special sandals which will earth you automatically and equally possible to buy bed sheets which either plug into earth systems in the house or can be attached to copper rods driven into the ground to earth your body and pick up the earth's natural rhythms whilst sleeping.

<u>Earthing</u>

We continually build up and discharge static electricity from our bodies. This is largely contributed by the high levels of friction in our environment (carpets, furniture, plastic accoutrements and so forth).

You will often note that getting down from your car after a long journey you get a bit of a shock when you earth the static charge that's built up or similarly when you walk across woollen or manmade fibre carpets and touch a door knob which sometimes gives you a shock.

Your body is subjected to countervailing flows of electromagnetism all the time, and the method by which you can harness this energy (and in some circumstances protect yourself against it) in order to improve your health and slow down the ageing process is by taking regular amount of Vitamin C. This improves the conductivity of your entire system and helps maintain full, good health.

MY DAILY DOSAGES.

1. I take between 5 and 10 grams (1,000 milligram tablets) of Vitamin C as ascorbic acid with citrus bioflavonoids and rosehips which come in the same tablet. (This is my maintenance dose).
2. I also take 400 milligram of turmeric twice a day
3. Two 1000 milligram linseed vegetable pods
4. 400 international units of Vitamin E mixed tocopherols
5. 50 pica-grams of selenium
6. One Vitamin B complex tablet
7. One 5,000 international unit capsule of Vitamin D3 and Vitamin K2 combined,
8. 150 milligram of magnesium,
9. 15 milligram of zinc with copper
10. Two drops of Lugol's iodine daily in a small glass of water before breakfast
11. I also take one high-quality vegetable sourced multivitamin each day
12. 120 milligram coenzyme Q10 capsule.
13. 5 x 250mg capsules of potentised charcoal C_{60} capsules last thing at night with water.

14. I work with negative ionizers beside my bed, on my desk and in my sitting-room.
15. I try and walk barefoot at least a mile a day through the countryside so as to absorb the maximum air energy available and thoroughly earth my systems. I also wear a magnetic bracelet.
16. I take ½ a teaspoon of sodium bicarbonate dissolved in a pint of water every morning first thing, before a cup of lemon tea. This gets me off to a good start every day and helps keep my system slightly alkaline.

NOTE: These are spread throughout the day so as not to over-alkalize my system at any one time.

Also, I have a complete break from all of the above for a few days every month to give my system a 'rest'.

The reason that I take this complex of vitamins and minerals is that they all contribute to protecting me from Cancer.

Now you might think that you don't want to take all these but consider that we live in an increasingly poisoned environment stiff with carcinogens, neurotoxins and endocrine disrupters. Your body needs all the help it can get and you should, at least, take Vitamin C.

I detail all the research which supports this assertion in my book *"**The Answer to Cancer**"* ISBN 978-0-9532407-5-3 available via Amazon online.

CONCLUSION

My father, and millions like him, died unnecessarily. His early death left my mother devastated and she never fully recovered. My brother and I grew up without a father and struggled to maintain that balance in our lives which is usually contributed by two parents. The fact that the link between Vitamin C deficiency and heart disease wasn't discovered until the late 1940s was tragic for us. However, the fact that this cure for heart disease is still relatively (almost completely) unknown is unforgiveable and the pharmaceutical industry with the medical profession bear responsibility for millions of avoidable deaths up to the present day.

In this book I have tried to reference a substantial body of scientifically proven research to persuade you to the point of view that taking large quantities of Vitamin C can save your life and extend your life. I sincerely hope that you'll take this to heart and take responsibility for your own health at a time when clearly the powers that be, with their vested interests, will not!

More information will be made available on my seminars and details of these can be found at http://www.keithfoster.co.uk. Meantime, I wish you the very best of health.

References / Sources

Nobel laureates

1. PAULING Dr. Linus. Twice Nobel Prize winner 1980's. *The role of Vitamin C as a powerful anti-cholesterol agent.*

2. SZENT-GYORGYI Albert. Discovered Vitamin C in 1932 and recommended use of Iodine. He received the Nobel Prize in Medicine in 1937.

3. WARBURG Otto, MD. Nobel Prize 1931 – *Research on respiratory enzymes certain vitamins and minerals that the body require for the utilization of oxygen in the cells.*

Other Sources

1. APPLEWHITE Roger. Electrical Engineer. *The effect of Grounding reduces Impact of EM Fields on Body.*

2. BATMANGHELIDJ Dr F. *Your Bodies Many Cries for Water*   ISBN 978-0970245885

3. BECKER Robert O. MD and Gary Selden. *The Body Electric*   ISBN 0-688-06971-1.

4. BROWNSTEIN Dr David M.D. *Iodine and Why You Need It.*   ISBN 978-0-9660882-3-6

5. CAMERON Ewan and Linus Pauling *Cancer and Vitamin C*   ISBN 0-446-97735-7.

6. CHERASKIN Dr Emanuel. Dr W. Marshall, Dr Ringsdorf Jr., and Dr Emily L. Sisley. *The Vitamin C Connection.* ISBN 0-7225-0908-1.

7. CLINTON Ober and Stephen T. Sinatra M.D. *Earthing.* ISBN 978-1-59120-283-7

8. DANLEY Tom. NASA Consultant and Acoustic Engineer, has identified 4 frequencies which form an F# chord Encyclopaedia Britannica – *Definition of Power Function in Resonance.*

9. DICKENSON Donald, PhD. *How to Fortify your Immune System* ISBN 0-85140-633-5.

10. DUBROV Prof. Alexander. Russian Scientist. Confirms support for Field and Resonance Concepts.

11. DURRANT-PEATFIELD Dr Barry, MBBS LRCP MRCS. Medical advisor to Thyroid UK. *Fluoride and its effects on the thyroid production of hormones controlling appetite.*

12. FEYNMAN Richard. Nobel Prize Physicist (1965) describes earth's subtle energies.

13. FOSTER Keith, FLS. *Harmonic Power Parts II – VI* (Sagax Publishing 2015) ISBN 978-0-9532407-7-0.

14. FRASSETTO Dr Lynda. (1996) University of California, San Francisco. Paper on *Bicarbonate levels in human blood vary with age.*

15. FULLER Buckminster, Architect. Carbon fullerenes are named after the Geodesic Dome he designed.

16. GHALY Dr Morris. (2004) Journal of Complementary Medicine. *Earthing During Sleep Resynchronises Cortisol Secretion During Sleep.* ISBN 978-0-9660882-3-6.

17. GROSS L. (1964). *Biological Effects of Magnetic Fields*, Vol. 1, Plenum Press, New York

18. McCance & Widdowson *The Composition of Foods*, 1978 – 2002.

19. NAKAGAWA Dr. The Isuzu Hospital, Tokyo, Japan *"Magnetic Field Deficiency Syndrome and Magnetic Treatment"*

20. OKAI Dr Kyorin. University, Japan. *Life Prolonging Attributes of Magnetic Fields.*

21. ROSS Dr William. (1999) Article in Podiatry Management against wearing shoes. Also (1997) Footwear News. *Study of nerve endings on foot.*

22. SIRCUS Dr. Mark. *Sodium Bicarbonate – Natures Unique First Aid Remedy.* ISBN 978-0-7570-0394-3.

23. SOYKA Fred with Alan Edmonds, *The Ion Effect* ISBN 0-553-12866-3.

24. STONE Dr Irwin. (published in 1980's) *"Scurvy" the most misunderstood epidemic disease in the 20th century.*

25. STONE I. *The genetics of scurvy and the cancer problem.* J. Orthomolecular Psychiatry Vol 5, No. 3, 183-190, 1976.

26. VERKEEK Dr R. BSc MSc DIC PHD, Executive and Scientific Director, The Alliance for Natural Health. *The Pros and Cons of water chlorination.*

27. British Medical Journal 24thMarch 2006. Reviewing 96 trials including 44 with supplements and with ALA (alpha linoleic acid) from plants; the remainder being fish oils, found no evidence to a clear benefit from Omega 3 fats on health.

28. British Medical Journal, 7th April 2005; BMJ 2005;330:853 *No Sweet Surrender,* (article on sugar).

29. Canadian Journal of Surgery (1993); *Iodine relieves symptoms of fibrocystic breast disease in 70% of patients.*

30. The Cambridge International Institute for Medical Science. Paper on *Omega-3 and Omega-6 also fish oils.*

31. US Food & Drug Admin, Dept. of Health & Human Resources, FDA, Poisonous Plant Database, March 2006 Revision. 288 *Records of Soy*

CPSIA information can be obtained
at www.ICGtesting.com
Printed in the USA
LVOW12s0340090817
544325LV00001B/92/P